Power of Love

21 Winning Ways to Attract Your Ideal Partner

Published in 2010 by

Fast Forward Publishing

London UK

ISBN: 978-1-4466-5881-9

Cover photo: © thaut images- fotolia.com

Printed by www.Lulu.com

This book is dedicated in love to all my past relationships, and Andy my husband, for helping to show me who I am

Contents

21 Winning Ways to Attract Your Ideal Partner

Love: A Path to Wholeness

We read and write novels and poems about it. We direct and watch films and plays about it. We make music, write and listen to songs about it. We talk about it, and from our youth to our old age we seek it. We've even created a whole language to describe how we feel about it.

LOVE.

It would seem we all yearn for this experience, yet what actually is this crazy thing we call love? Why do we need it and more importantly, how and where do we find it?

Without understanding fully what it is we seek when we look for love, we have created a myth of romantic fantasy that has its origin in fairy stories told to us from childhood, in which princesses are woken up from evil spells by a kiss and where Prince Charming saves Cinderella from a life of hate and drudgery transporting her to one of adoration and luxury.

We have also built up huge expectations on how love should make us feel when we do find it. And for many people those initial feelings known as the period of romantic love can bring about overwhelming emotions from feeling alive and extremely happy to feeling out of control and vulnerable.

The truth is that although you and I want love, we surely don't consciously choose 'it', for when love happens it is often 'out of the blue' or at the very least takes us by surprise. We also have little or no control as to how long those exuberant feelings of love last and indeed for some people falling in and out of love are frequent occurrences throughout their adult life.

We confirm that love 'happens' to us when we say we have 'fallen in love', for we are indicating a behaviour in which we have no choice, as we literally 'fall into it'. So if falling in love with someone is something that happens to us without conscious thought, what happens to us when we 'fall in love' and more importantly how do we know we've found the right person to fall in love with?

The first indication that a person experiences when they fall in love is that they have a compelling urge to be with the other person. They experience strong emotions, so strong in fact are these feelings that they can overwhelm rational thought and judgment, hence the terms "head over heels" and "heart ruling head". Some people even experience "love at first sight" whilst others may come to it over time. Make no mistake, love and relationships in general, are emotional and complicated and deep seated within your subconscious mind. Regardless to what you and I might think, attraction to another isn't about personal choice, for our subconscious minds have their own agenda when it comes to falling in love.

Romantic love is full of fantasies conjuring up images of knights in shining armor and going off with arms linked together into the sunset, living happily ever after. Just when the story gets interesting and you want to know what happens next, it abruptly ends and you are left wondering. Perhaps it was intentional... After all once those heady feelings of being "in love" pass and you come back to reality with a bump and realize that your prince or princess is not so perfect after all, the story would have to have a different ending.

Unlike the fairy tales, the story of true love gets really gets interesting. And it's here when the story of your own emotional growth really starts to go up a notch, for in order to achieve long lasting, healthy, loving relationships we must dispel the myth that the state of romantic love lasts forever.

Romantic love is a temporary event; therefore enjoy it whilst it lasts, as sooner or later you will feel disappointment with your partner. Where once you felt comfortable around him or her, you will inevitably become irritated or frustrated, little things that you excused or were blinded to suddenly become visible, and those 'high' feelings, loss of appetite, and sleep wear off sooner or later as you crash back to earth.

But *please* don't panic because it doesn't mean you don't love your partner any more. It is meant to be this way. There are very good reasons for 'coming back to earth', and it is all due to your subconscious mind taking you on to the next stage in your relationship and your own personal growth. And let's face it, your body just can't sustain those overwhelming emotions every day for the rest of your life, and at the risk of sounding a party pooper, those wonderful, elated emotions happen because of chemicals that your body releases in response to your subconscious attraction to the other person.

These natural chemicals are related to the amphetamine drug group, the main ones being phenyl ethylamine and dopamine and have a similar affect as endorphins. They increase your energy level and your sexual desire, reduce your appetite and disrupt your sleep patterns and have a positive effect on your mental attitude.

The reason why your brain releases these chemicals is because your subconscious mind believes it has found the person who is able to help you become whole.

Like the swans on the front cover of this book, most of us look for a mate for life. But unlike animals, who instinctively select a mate on the basis of their ability to survive and breeding potential, humans are much more complex. Whilst health, fitness and beauty are considerations, humans want to form an emotional attachment or bond to their mate to enable them to become whole. Again we can see an expression of this need in our language, for someone might say "I can't live without him or her", "he/she completes me" and "I feel whole now we are together". We certainly don't seek love with the thought of divorce or separation. Our intention is that love should last forever.

So why do we need to feel whole. In Freudian terms it is quite simply to overcome death. In feeling whole we can feel safe, secure and intact. The fear of death is conquered as we create images of love being eternal, lasting forever.

Since birth your subconscious is compelled to restore the feeling of wholeness that you had when you were born. Prior to birth you had no awareness of anything other than yourself. You were complete, as if you were your within your own world. This is how you entered the world. As you started to develop, you made demands on the world around you; you learnt how to get your needs met. For example, if you were hungry, you would cry and your mother (or other caregiver) would feed you. Sometimes your needs were unmet, or didn't happen immediately and subsequently you began to realize that you were dependent on others to meet those needs. As you grew, you began to understand that you were not complete and self-sufficient, creating a feeling of insecurity deep in your subconscious. This unrest is what drives your subconscious, as its primary goal is to reach wholeness, and subsequently safety.

It is likely that as you grew up you also experienced emotional wounding. Childhood hurts, fears and self-limiting beliefs block your emotional growth. As well as your subconscious striving to meet unmet needs from early childhood, it also wants to heal those early wounds, as it is necessary in order to reach wholeness.

Your subconscious does this by looking for a person who has similar traits of your parents or caregivers, assuming that those qualities are essential to meet your needs and continue your growth. Once it's recognized these traits in another person, it's likely you'll feel a sudden inexplicable attraction to them. When this happens, some people experience a feeling of 'completeness' whilst others may feel that there is something familiar about the other person, like they've 'known' them all their life almost as though they have just been waiting for them to appear. This is because your mind 'sees' your parent or caregiver in this person.

Don't just take my word for this. Write out a list of at least 10 positive and 10 negative personality traits for each parent or caregiver. Then reflect back on past relationships and write another list of positive and negative traits. When finished compare your lists and notice familiar patterns and similar traits. Quite commonly you'll find traits from one parent or caregiver is more evident than the other in your choice of partners. This is no accident.

Once you've found that person who has similarities or traits from your early caregivers, your mind triggers the release of those feel-good chemicals I mentioned earlier and well, off goes the fireworks! Its celebration time and you feel wonderful.

After a while your subconscious realizes that the person you've met is not meeting those unmet needs from childhood, and consequently your brain body releases less of these feel good chemicals.

At this stage disappointment can set in and even conflict can occur. When this happens it is important to work on your own emotions and find out what it is from your past that is causing this distress, otherwise the relationship inevitably deteriorates. Some people at this stage believe their initial judgment on choosing their partner was wrong, and that they haven't found Mr. or Mrs. Right after all. Subsequently, they might even finish the relationship and unfortunately take all their baggage (their unresolved unmet needs from the past) and take them directly into their next relationship, repeating this cycle over and over again until your subconscious mind resolves these issues once and for all.

So, if you are looking for that feeling of romantic love to last forever, then I'm sorry to say, you are going to be disappointed. However, it is important to understand that romantic love is the first stage of a relationship, and whilst it is exciting and wonderful, if we are serious about wanting a truly, loving, supportive, satisfying and fulfilling relationship to grow from it, then we have to work on ourselves first. And the best time is before you have a relationship. If you can work on resolving your childhood wounds before you commit to someone, you will not be as 'needy' and demanding in a relationship and when you do meet someone, you will be more aware of why you may expect more from the other person than he or she can give.

Relationships are a not only a beautiful gift in our lives that can bring us so much pleasure, but that they are also the living feedback that we need to listen to carefully, which will enable us to grow and mature fully into the person we are meant to become.

If you want to find the ideal partner or soul mate for you to share a fulfilling, intimate, supportive and loving relationship, then this booklet will help you start the process. Each tip will guide you through how you can avoid the mistakes, snares and pitfalls that are commonly and unwittingly made and prepare you to meet your soul mate.

Tip #1 Stop Looking For the Perfect Partner

"We begin to love not by finding a perfect person, but by learning to see an imperfect person perfectly."
Source Unknown.

When looking for love, many people look for the perfect person, believing there is such a person 'out there' waiting to be discovered. It's my belief that there is a danger in thinking this way, as firstly, you run the risk of never meeting "Mr. or Miss Perfect, and may have missed your ideal soul mate because you've been too specific in your selection, and secondly, it's highly likely that once you've settled down with Mr. or Miss Perfect, you start to find out that he/she isn't so perfect after all, and, if you're not careful could end up believing you've made a mistake, and consequently end the relationship.

If you've been looking or are currently looking for *the* perfect partner I can guarantee you will eventually be disappointed as no such person exists. You'd simply be wasting your time and energy as you will be looking forever and will never be satisfied because every time you discover a fault you will be looking elsewhere (if you've any doubts about this just take a look around you).

You may have narrowed down a list of qualities that you want, and even if he or she ticks all the right boxes, pretty soon you'll find there is something that you don't like about them, or a behaviour that irritates you. So the best thing to do is to dispense with the idea immediately that there is a perfect partner out there waiting to be discovered.

However, there is good news, it is possible to discover the ideal partner for **you**, someone who matches the hidden criteria *you* have subconsciously created, who possesses the qualities *you* need that will enable *you* to grow emotionally and spiritually. But for you to be successful at attracting this person to you, you have to know who *you* are and to do this you will need to find out what's on your hidden list of criteria! Remember emotional attraction is subconscious.

So instead of seeking the "perfect" partner into your life, you need to seek a partner who is right for you and finding this person is only part of the process, as in order to find the ideal mate, you have to **become** the ideal mate. That's right, **you** need to be willing to change, and grow into the person who you are destined to be. You will need to delve into your subconscious and uncover **who** you are, and what you need from a relationship.

Doing this doesn't have to be difficult, you can easily learn skills that can help you to access your inner resources which will assist you in building a satisfying, successful relationship. The first step then is to make a commitment and form an intention now to further your own self-growth.

Tip #2 Never Ever Settle for 2nd Best

"I love you not only for what you are, but for what I am when I am with you. I love you not only for what you have made of yourself, but for what you are making of me. I love you for the part of me that you bring out. "

- Elizabeth Barrett Browning

There can be an enormous amount of pressure these days to be in a relationship. Even though times have changed, and it is now more socially acceptable to be single, there is still the "social norm" to *"tie the knot"* and "settle down" with one partner. One of our basic emotional needs is to feel secure, and have a sense of belonging whether it's to a family, or even a peer group. These groups help us to feel accepted and safe. Even if we like to be different, we will still gravitate towards like-minded people to seek and enjoy their approval.

Some people feel uncomfortable if they don't fit into cultural social norms. These people may feel there is something about themselves that is unacceptable, or even unlikable. Their feelings may even tap into an inner belief that they feel undeserving of a healthy, happy and fulfilling relationship, and for some people this can mean any relationship is better than no relationship.

If this resonates with you, be careful. The solution does not lie in accepting any relationship. The danger in thinking this way can leave you vulnerable and at risk of entering a relationship for all the wrong reasons, and in the worse case scenario end up being with a person not ideally suited to you. Despite inevitably causing great unhappiness to you both, this can also reinforce a low self-esteem, leading you to liking yourself even less than you did to start with. So make sure your desire to be in a relationship is not about a need to feel better about yourself.

Resist pressure and take the time you need to find out what it is you truly desire and need from a relationship before you act – after all it's the rest of your life we are talking about, and settling for second best in a relationship is a bit like wearing a new pair of boots a size too small. Even though you may look good in them, they just don't fit right, are extremely uncomfortable and painful, and usually end up being thrown out at the end of the day.

Tip # 3 Thinking You Can Change Your Partner

"When you like someone, you like them in spite of their faults. When you love someone, you love them with their faults. "

- Elizabeth Cameron

Another reason someone might be in a relationship with someone they are not happy with, is the belief that they can change them into the person they want them to be. A lot of people believe it is mainly women that do this, but men equally are guilty. Usually men are more explicit, using control, either verbally or physically, whilst women are more subtle and more manipulative. However, both aim to achieve the same thing – that is changing their partner to be the person they want to be.

One of the main reasons as to why some people want to do this, goes back again to our basic need for emotional security. Rather than deal with their own insecurity, (which could mean dealing with painful memories) there is the mistaken belief that if the person they are with changes then they will feel more secure. And if they can be instrumental in bringing about those changes in him/her without experiencing the anxiety and possibly fear of dealing with their own insecurities, then all the better!

How untrue this is! Trying to change your partner is a bit like redecorating your neighbours' house without their permission. You have no business and no right to be there, and they will eventually resent you. You see people will consistently be who they are, so it is likely that any change you try to impose on another will meet resistance and be rejected, openly or covertly.

You simply cannot change someone else. You can only change yourself. Stop deceiving yourself that you can change someone, and instead put your energy into looking at yourself and dealing with what it is that leaves you feeling insecure. Once you feel more confident within yourself, your attitude, behaviour and responses to others will change and consequently so will your partners' as he/she will not re-act to you in the same way. By dealing with your own issues you will create a relationship where you are not relying on your partner to make you feel secure. That feeling will come from inside yourself. Remember you can only change what **you** own – take responsibility for yourself.

Tip # 4 Take Responsibility for Yourself

"Love is shown in your deeds, not in your words."

-- Fr. Jerome Cummings

Stop blaming others and start taking responsibility for yourself, for your life, and for your feelings and attitudes. In thinking about your relationships, it's important to remember to take 100% responsibility for who you are today. Quite often, people emerge from a broken relationship placing all the blame for the break up on to the other person, or onto circumstances, or even on to other people. You've heard the phrase 'it takes two to tango', and there are always 2 sides to every story.

A few years back a good friend of mine was totally devastated when her husband left her with 4 children and a Dear John letter. Understandably she was felt extremely hurt and angry with him. They never got back together and he met someone else. She however continued to fuel her anger and pain of rejection, and saw herself as a victim becoming bitter and judgemental. At no time did she ask herself why her marriage had ended. She blamed him for everything and refused to accept responsibility for not picking up on the warning signs and early communication he would have sent her, telling her that things were not right in their relationship. Had she done so, who knows what would have happened, and the outcome may have been completely different.

You and you alone are responsible for your feelings, and no one can *make* you feel anything. Only you can choose how to feel, and the good news is that you can learn to change your feelings through making positive choices.

For many years I worked with women and men where domestic violence was a frequent occurrence in their relationship. Often a perpetrator would say "she/he made me so angry" or "he/she deserved it" and I've even heard "it wasn't me, something took over inside, and made me do it". But abdication of personal responsibility was not just from the person who committed the abuse. Many victims would say "I can't leave him/her" "I have no choice" and "I asked for it".

Now obviously it's not acceptable to abuse another person, but the flip side is that if you accept abuse, you have to take responsibility for it, since no one but you allows yourself to be abused simply by still being around them. In doing this you are giving your partner unspoken permission to carry on being abusive. If you find yourself with an abusive partner, I urge you to take action. The only way is to find the strength to move on from them so that you can find the right person. I am not saying this is easy, and you may need to draw support from others, but inevitably it's the only way.

Taking responsibility means dealing with unfinished business, whether this is finishing off a practical task or if you have offended someone. Take responsibility, apologise and if it is possible and appropriate make an intention to put things right. You will find that as you take more responsibility for your life, behaviour and emotions, you become elevated to a higher place, where you will feel at peace with yourself knowing that you have done all that you can.

If you are blaming another person, or others, you will only attract to you a person who mirrors yourself, and when we are in judgement of another it is usually because there is something about that person that is true about ourselves. Examine carefully those who you struggle with and find the comparison in yourself. Be honest and truthful. By taking responsibility for yourself, and working on transforming your own negative qualities into positive attributes, you will attract a person to you who shares those same qualities and values.

Tip # 5 Stop Thinking About How Lonely You Feel

"If you want to be loved, be lovable"

- Ovid

A lot of people who long for a fulfilling, loving relationship often focus on how lonely they feel, not having someone they can intimately share with. In a lot of cases these people dwell too much on their loneliness, and may even talk about how hard it is living on their own, hardly spending any time at all talking about the relationship they would like to have one day. They may even isolate themselves from others spending time alone at home. Face facts, if you hide yourself away from the flow of life how on earth will you meet anyone. You will miss so many opportunities of meeting new people and making friends and may be even miss meeting your ideal partner.

There is another problem too. One of the most powerful of the universal laws is the law of attraction. What this means in simple terms is that we attract to us more of what we think and feel. It works on the notion that our minds are like magnets, and our thoughts and feelings are forms of energy. We send out this energy, which are called vibrations or 'vibes' into the universe around us, which in turn attracts back to us more of the same. So if your thoughts are focused on how lonely you feel, this message is being transmitted outside of you, and consequently you will attract even more loneliness to your life. This, of course, is entirely the wrong message to send if you want to attract a loving partner and fulfilling relationship into your life.

Tip # 6 Let Go and Move On

"Those who do not know how to weep with their whole heart do not know how to laugh either."

- Golda Meir

Some people find it incredibly hard to move on from past relationships and I've come across many people whose topic of conversations always end with them talking about a previous partner and going over what went wrong. It's like they're stuck, and in a lot of cases it's true, because these people are holding themselves as victims to the past. I am not saying here that it is not important to review things when we feel something has gone wrong in our life, for its necessary to learn from these situations to avoid repeating them in the future. Nor am I saying you should bury emotions such as feeling hurt, angry or depressed. But to acknowledge those emotions and deal with them and not keep analyzing them.

Emotions are just energy. They are essentially our feedback as to how things are with us. They tell us when things are not okay. To illustrate what I mean, consider this scenario. If you put your hand in a fire, you will feel physical pain which warns you to pull your hand away otherwise it will burn. Likewise if your emotion is fear or guilt, it is a warning that things are not right, and you need to take appropriate action.

You and I need to listen to our emotions and express them in some way, in doing this we are not blocking or suppressing the energy flow. For instance if you are hurting and feel angry, it is important to accept that pain and anger to be expressed in a safe way. Just as we have to listen to our bodies, in the same way we need to listen to our emotions. Once we've allowed ourselves to accept and voiced our feelings, it becomes easier to release them.

Many people these days numb out and avoid their feelings by turning externally to food, alcohol, drugs, gambling, and even sport activities and work. This is not the answer. Your feelings are there for a reason and need to be acknowledged. Avoiding or numbing out your feelings is a bit like burying a man alive, he is always scratching to get to the surface. Trust me, your feelings will not go away, unless you acknowledge them, they are still there inside you and your subconscious mind will remind you of them at any opportunity.

There are a number of different techniques you can apply that will enable you to acknowledge, accept and express these emotions, and then let them go, allowing you to move up the emotional scale to a more positive feeling. If you need to have a good cry, or punch a pillowcase, and when you've done, do something you enjoy doing, even if it's just stroking the cat. Get support to help you through this if you need to. Doing nothing and obsessing about situations and blaming others for their cause is not the way forward and as I stated earlier will only attract to you more of the same for the future.

So if you find yourself falling in this trap, work towards a healthy state of mind and wellbeing by choosing to consider that all past difficult relationships are preparation for true love. Accept them as an important part of your life and learn to appreciate those people because they have taught you what you don't want from a relationship. Find a way to express gratitude for even those toughest lessons that you've learned. Release yourself spiritually from the past by forgiving them and thanking them through prayer or meditation for their role in an important and instructive part of your life journey and then let them go.

Once you've freed that space in your heart that has been occupied by a previous relationship, you'll find you have created space for a new love, confident in knowing more clearly what it is that you want in your relationship.

Tip # 7 Throw Out Your Rubbish

"You have to fall in love with yourself before anyone will fall in love with you. Define yourself by who you are and not who you're with"

- Kathleen Marvelli

This is a really important tip. Imagine for a moment that all of us were born perfect but with a blank sheet of paper, and as we grew up, other people close to us wrote on that piece of paper their comments, negative and positive, about us. We also added to that paper, by writing down our experiences of events throughout childhood, and as a result, this piece of paper contains all the beliefs and values that we hold about ourselves and the world around us and it is stored within the very core of our being.

As adults we make reference to this piece of paper in our everyday life. That is every event, every experience that you and I have, and how we feel about ourselves at any given moment. All of us subconsciously refer back to our core values and beliefs. It is therefore essential in finding the right partner for you, that you stop looking on the outside, and instead look inside yourself and work on those beliefs you have about yourself that limit your life, or have negative connotations for you. Remember for the most part they are mistaken beliefs made by others that you have made your own.

True love is not just about romance, and great sex. When you meet someone and fall in love, you eventually have to decide whether you want a real, lasting, relationship with that person, warts and all, or whether you want to continue looking for that elusive "perfect" partner all over again. If you decide to look elsewhere, you still have to take your baggage with you into the next relationship and so on. That baggage will go with you no matter who you are with and where you go, until you decide to dump it for good.

Once you commit and embark on a journey of self-awareness and discovery you will find you will naturally attract to you a person who is also interested in self-growth and who shares similar values and who like you, wants a strong equal loving and supportive relationship.

Tip # 8 Quit Punishing Yourself

"Any fact facing us is not as important as our attitude toward it, for that determines our success or failure."

- Norman Vincent Peale

As mentioned previously, over time and from an early age we develop self-limiting beliefs about ourselves. A common belief is "I'm not good enough at ……" This belief usually stems from childhood, where someone, perhaps in this case at teacher or a parent has said "you're no good at ….. " Or "you're bad at ……" Consequently the mistaken belief develops and the adult person goes around thinking they are useless at – whatever it is – and doesn't have the confidence to try any more.

This is just one example of a self-limiting belief. Remember these are mistaken beliefs that other people have made, that you hold to be true, and manifest themselves in self-criticism, and by continuing to believe them, your confidence and self-esteem will be affected.

Another mistaken belief we have is that if we use the tools learned in our childhood to get what we want, we will be successful at getting our needs met in our relationship. I am referring here to the tactics we used as children, such as screaming the house down, temper tantrums, mood swings, sulkiness and withdrawal. They may have worked with our parents, but our partners are not our early caregivers, and will respond in an entirely different way. Lay down these emotional weapons as the only person you are punishing is yourself.

In doing nothing about these negative beliefs, you are doing nothing about making life better and more fulfilling for yourself. Only you have the responsibility for yourself. Start by becoming aware of your behaviour and responses and make connections with your past by looking for patterns of similar behaviour responses. Learn to understand why you feel the way you do about a situation and what triggers off your reactions.

When you nurture yourself, you are affirming to the world that you are an okay person, where mistakes are held as a learning experience, where there is no such thing as failure just growth. If you feel you have negative beliefs about yourself that block you from doing the things you want to do in life and want to learn how you can let go of those self-limiting thoughts and feelings, make an intention today to seek counselling, self-help books, therapy or attend a self-growth workshop. To help you get started I have listed some resources at the back of this book

Once you let go of those self-limiting beliefs, you will create a new energy, and become a person who attracts people to like who you are, and not someone you are pretending to be. If you want to receive love you must learn how to accept love.

After all how can you expect someone to love you, when you don't love yourself?

Tip # 9 Embrace Singledom

"If you are single, eliminate the thought that something is lacking and just live each day joyfully"

- Jonathan Lockwood Huie

Some people hate being single, and imagine that when they finally find "The One" *then* life will be complete, they will be finally happy and start living. This is simply not true!

Every one of us should live life to the full and enjoy the present moment, regardless of whether we are in a relationship or not. Happiness is about appreciation. The quickest way to feel happy is to focus on something that you appreciate. The more things you can appreciate the happier you become. A good tip here is to start a gratitude journal and each day write down all the things that you feel grateful for. Shift your focus on these things and something spiritual starts to happen as you feel more content with your life. Secondly, time is our most valuable asset - once it's gone it's gone forever. If you're constantly thinking "I'll be happy when…." You are missing out on today and all that life offers you, you simply cannot put your life on hold.

Furthermore, if you are living life to the full it is your zest for life that will attract your ideal partner or soul mate to you. Being authentic and the person who you are is how he or she will recognise you. For just as you are subconsciously seeking your ideal partner, the same thing is happening to him or her. Believe it, he or she is already looking for you. So make sure you are true to yourself so that he/she can easily recognize you.

Honour the state of not yet having a mate and enjoy life. Go out with friends, and spend time developing skills, nurturing interests, and perhaps traveling and having adventures. Create the life you want to lead and enjoy it.

You are in the ideal situation to have the time and commitment to focus on your own personal development. Define what you want in all arenas of your life, not just relationships, such as career choice or profession, health and leisure goals.

Tip # 10 Be True to Yourself

"There is no disguise which can hide love for long where it exists, or simulate it where it does not."

- Duc de la Rochefoucauld

Some people go to extra-ordinary lengths in order to attract a partner. These can include spending huge amounts of time and money on improving our physique and fitness by attending a gym and going on special diets, maybe even spending a fortune on exterior assets and status symbols such as cars, clothes, accessories, perfumes, toiletries, and beauty products, all to improve our image. But there are also less obvious ones; such as entering a sexual relationship before you are ready to or going the extra mile all the time just to impress. Other common examples are pretending to have the same interests, or even lying about your current situation and circumstances and appearing more emotionally healthy than you actually are.

So why are we tempted to impress and pretend to be someone we're not? One of the main reasons why many people go to such lengths is because they fear rejection. This fear is based on the belief that if a prospective partner found out who they really was they might not like them.

Remember, you don't have to act or pretend to be someone you're not for someone to like you. Just be yourself and stop seeking approval. There is simply no point in pretending otherwise, because people will consistently be the person they are which is why just changing your behaviour and habits are so difficult. You will not be able to keep it up indefinitely and in the long-term the truth will out, and by then the chances are you will have lost them anyway. You only have to think of how unsuccessful New Year Resolutions if you need proof of this.

If you find yourself trying to impress a "potential" partner by being someone you're not or by telling lies about yourself then I urge you to STOP! You won't gain a thing and you certainly won't fool anyone other than yourself. Stop kidding yourself and ask yourself what it is that you are afraid of. Overcome the fear by being the real you.

Tip # 11 Learn That It Is Not Just About You

"Love is that condition in which the happiness of another person is essential to your own"

– Robert Heinlein

Someone once said that no man is an island. If you want to have a successful relationship, then you have to learn that it is not just about you. There is no such thing as a total and absolute truth; as everyone has their own perspective based on their personal experience. In making a relationship work, it's important to learn to be able to see things from the other persons' perspective, and sometimes that means you have to shift position to understand more fully. Listen carefully to what the other person is saying and empathise with their experience of life, so that you can fully understand where they are coming from and why they might feel things differently to you. If necessary check out with the other person that you've understood correctly. Stop listening to your own hurts and wounds and see things from another perspective first before you express your opinion.

Any change to your life has a ripple effect, especially on others who are close to you. Before starting a relationship, it's also worth thinking about what disruption elsewhere may occur, and working out how you will deal with that once you are in the relationship. For example, if you have young children from a previous relationship, it's essential that you consider their needs as a priority. Think about how you would see your new partner within the family relationship, and the contact you have with your ex-partner. Other people in your life may also be affected and need re-assuring, so it is important that you still include them in your life, talking with them honestly about what you want for your future.

As well as other people, it is necessary to also consider the circumstances and context of your relationship which may not be ideal and if this is the case you may need to give a lot of careful thought. Geographic distances, employment situation, marital status, religious and cultural differences to name a few can all create additional tensions in any relationship, so look where disruptions may present themselves and plan how you will deal with them, always acting with integrity, truth and honesty.

Tip # 12 Mirror, Mirror on the Wall...

Love built on beauty, soon as beauty, dies."
~ John Donne

A mistake a lot of people make when thinking about their ideal partner is that they focus on the outside image and not on the inner qualities. You see examples of this all the time in dating columns in newspapers and on matchmaking sites on the internet, and in personal ads such as 'tall, handsome body builder, seek petite, attractive, blonde lady for lasting relationship.'

I am not saying there is anything wrong in being attracted to appearance, however, don't let it be the only criteria for choosing a partner. Appearances are only skin deep and it's what's under the surface that will tell whether a relationship will last or not.

In virtually every couple I meet in relationship counselling I ask each person this same question "what attracted you to your partner", and almost every time the replies are inner qualities; such as sense of humour, intelligence, solidness, etcetera, rarely have I heard replies regarding physical image as being a main attraction. This tells me that despite what we think we prefer, it is the inner qualities that our subconscious is seeking out in the other person, so it is essential we don't block this by being overly image conscious.

The truth here is that if you are looking for the ideal match for you, then you have to go beyond skin deep. You have to draw up a list of inner qualities that you want. It is these qualities your subconscious mind seeks and attracts to you. Physical image may bring about attraction, but attachment happens on emotional level based on inner qualities.

Tip # 13 Focus on What You Want From a Relationship

"As you think, you travel, and as you love, you attract. You are today where your thoughts have brought you; you will be tomorrow where your thoughts take you. "

~ James Allen

Napoleon Hill said "what the mind conceives and believes, it achieves" yoga experts tell us 'where your attention goes your energy flows" and the Law of attraction works on the principal "ask, believe and receive". Yet when I ask my clients to tell me what qualities they want in the partner of their dreams, almost without exception they give me a list of what they don't want in their partner.

Let me explain. When I asked a client of mine what qualities she wanted in her ideal partner, she presented me with this list:

"Someone who doesn't smoke or drink too much"

"Someone who doesn't waste money likes it's going out of fashion"

"Someone who is not abusive"

And when I asked what she wanted from a relationship, her reply was;

"No fighting" and "no jealousy"

This woman had a history of relationships where her previous partners drunk and smoked excessively, were irresponsible with money and were physically violent towards her. Therefore it was no mystery to understand why her choice was expressed in this way as she clearly was afraid of history repeating itself in a future relationship. She was very clear about what she didn't want, but was not able to clearly articulate what she did want, and her primary emotion was fear.

Furthermore, what she didn't realize was that by formulating a list like this she was in fact asking for more of the same. You can imagine her horror on hearing this.

We are all familiar with self-fulfilling prophecy, but how many people are aware of the process of how it works.

To understand how, it's important to know that our brains 'think' in pictures. This is why we call this part of our brain the imagination. A statement such as "no fighting" is negative, and our brains cannot receive the word 'no' as it is difficult to present this in picture format. Consequently, the brain receives the word 'fighting' and forms an image of this. So whereas my client was meaning 'no fighting' her brain actually received 'fighting' as a message. And it doesn't stop there, as in the case of this woman, fighting triggered within her the emotion of fear which increased her negative energy vibrations. According to the law of attraction, we get more of what we focus on. The result was that this woman was attracting to her the very thing that she didn't want.

It is therefore absolutely vital for success to envision your ideal relationship always in the positive, and here's how to do it. Write down a list of all the qualities that you would like in your partner, and what you'd describe as a deeply fulfilling love relationship, making sure you have reframed any don't wants into positive statements – for example my client could have reframed her statements to;

"A person who has self-control"

"Someone who is respectful and considerate"

"A secure relationship built on trust"

Once you've made your list of positive statements visualize each one making sure that the image is representative of what you've written down, and correct any that needs amending, so it is all written in the positive.

Tip # 14 Imagine Your Ideal Relationship

"Love is the triumph of imagination over intelligence."

~ H. L. Mencken

Visualization is one of the most powerful tools you can use to bring to you the things you want out of life, and that includes attracting the right person to you. There is so much proof that visualization really works – from scientific research to testimonies from successful people, and the great thing is that you can visualize virtually anywhere, in any place at any time.

Remember your mind thinks in pictures and not in words, which means that if you are communicating with your subconscious just through words, then you'll have little chance of success. You have to 'speak' the same language otherwise it's a bit hit and miss, just like speaking English to someone who only speaks French – always communicate in pictures to you subconscious by using your imagination.

When you have composed your list of qualities that you want in your ideal partner, focus your mind and use your imagination to create a picture of what it would be like to be in loving, supportive, intimate, fulfilling relationship with this person. Let your mind conjure up images of your ideal relationship, how it would be, then allow yourself to imagine you are already there, letting yourself feel, see, and hear the experience as a whole as though it was really happening in the present moment.

For example, imagine "being held in the embrace of your loved one, feeling the warmth of their body, and breathing in their scent" and imagine how it feels to be listened to and supported.

Our thoughts on their own are powerful, yet when we add to them emotions the power is greatly amplified. Emotions carry enormous amounts of energy. You only have to think of the "atmosphere" you feel when you enter a room where the occupants have just had an argument to know what I mean. So when you are creating thoughts, add to the vision strong emotions by 'feeling' what it would be like, the energy you are creating will increase.

The energy you experience does two things; it gives your subconscious mind a powerful picture of what you want, and the greater the energy, the stronger the vibration you are sending into the universe.

For you to be successful, it is important to visualize daily your ideal relationship, and keep replaying this over and over as though you are in a movie. In doing so you are communicating with your subconscious sending out instructions to seek out the type of person you want and the relationship you desire. You may even find it helpful to draw a picture or symbol that represents that visualization, or create a vision board made up of cut out pictures that represent your idea of a perfect relationship. This has the effect of making it feel more 'real' and 'concrete', so that when someone asks you what it is you want, you will have clarity about your future. Images are a colourful vivid expression of what you want, so put your vision board in a place where you can see it frequently throughout the day, so that every time you look at it you are drawn back to your vision, and all the good feelings you have attached to it.

Tip # 15 Believe It Is For Real

"The best and most beautiful things in this world cannot be seen or even heard, but must be felt with the heart."

- Helen Kellar

Once you have a vision of what your ideal relationship looks and feels like, then the next step is to believe that he/she really exists and that your dream relationship will happen. Let's face it, if you don't believe your ideal partner exists then it's unlikely you will find him/her so it is important to change your beliefs. This is where affirmations can help you. Affirmations are a powerful tool to help you change your belief pattern from "I will never find the right person" to "I have found the ideal person"

A lot of people think affirmations are foolish and dismiss them, but all of us every day make affirmations whether we are consciously aware of it or not. Everything you say or think about is an affirmation. That includes all our self-talk, for example every time you say either out loud or to yourself "I'm not good enough at......." Or "I can't cope with…" You are affirming the belief that you are not good enough at 'whatever it is' and are telling your mind that you cannot cope.

Subconsciously through our affirming we are creating our life experience – moment by moment. These subconscious affirmations come from our inner beliefs, which may or may not be true, as many of them were constructed during our childhood. Some of these inner beliefs limit our hopes for the future and subsequently the subconscious negative affirmations we make sabotage any hopes we have for the future.

It's therefore essential to stop making unconscious automatic negative affirmations and start making positive conscious ones. Get in the habit of saying positive affirmations daily. Begin by composing a list of things that are not in your life at the moment but what you want to have. Remember focus on what you want NOT what you don't want. You may want to visit your qualities list you made earlier, or look at changing some of those limiting beliefs that you identified. Here are a couple of positive affirmations to get you started.

"I know that I deserve love and accept it now"

"I attract healthy and loving relationships"

There are 6 Golden Rules when creating an affirmation which are:

1 Always write in the present tense i.e. 'I am a loving, forgiving, generous person'

2 Make the statement positive i.e. 'I experience truth, love, and support in my relationship with my partner'

3 Always use action verbs i.e. 'I enjoy intimacy and great sex with my partner'

4 Keep each affirmation concise and brief i.e. 'I am the author of my life'

5 Use words in each affirmation that are meaningful to you..."I enjoy giving care and support to another"

6 As much as you'd like to never make affirmations for other people such as 'Tom loves cooking every night' only make affirmations for yourself.

Even if you are not in a relationship, your affirmations are about stating what you want in a relationship as though it was really happening in the here and now.

Once you've listed your affirmations, close your eyes and say each one of them out loud with passion. As you do so imagine that each affirmation is true and is happening in your life in the here and now. Engage all your senses to experience this reflection of the life you are now creating. Enjoy the images as you do so; remember your thoughts and your emotions are increasing in energy and vibration. The more positive you feel the better, and the more effective your affirmations will be.

Some people feel silly saying affirmations out loud everyday, particularly as they are about things that are yet to happen. If you feel this way, consider this, if you already believe that the right person with all the qualities you desire is out there, you would be attracting him/her already to you. But if that's not yet happened, and you don't want to risk attracting the "wrong" person to you, then try affirming that the right partner will show up sooner or later will happen, after all you have everything to gain. Remember, we get more of what we think about. Positive affirmations are a way of reprogramming your mind, challenging negative beliefs and fears and projecting positive happier thoughts.

I carry my affirmations with me all the time on a typed postcard, as well as having them written up on a whiteboard in my office. There are always moments during the day when I am able to visualise them and say them. Additionally it is really powerful to stand in from of your bathroom mirror (with the door locked) and say them out loud looking yourself in the eyes.

You may have heard some people say they have tried affirmations but it never changed anything for them. This is because of a very common mistake. For affirmations to be effective it is important that you repeat them at least twice a day, for at least a period of 30 days without a break. Scientific research has shown that the brain needs around 30 days to adapt itself to a new belief pattern. To remind yourself do as I do, write them on a card which you can carry around with you, or put them on post-it notes on a wall in your room, or if you've created a vision board, attach the list to it. Make sure you say your affirmations at least once a day every day for a minimum period of 30 days without a break. After then it should feel easier and you will find yourself naturally thinking your affirmations without effort. Try it and notice how much more positive you feel.

Tip # 16 Manifest your Ideal Person

"I have learned not to worry about love; But to honour its coming with all my heart" – Alice Walker

Okay I've suggested that you focus your thoughts on the qualities of the person you want to attract into your life, and I've explained how important it is to visualise your ideal relationship, *and* get in touch with how it feels to be in the images you've created. I've emphasised the importance of making daily affirmations to bring about a new belief pattern, and transforming your intentions for your relationship into realities. Now I'm going to share with you how this person, your ideal partner, will manifest in your life.

I mentioned earlier about thoughts and feelings having energy. Did you realise that every thought you have, every emotion you have is just energy. To prove my point, just think about that time when you walked into a room or situation where there has been an argument or heated debate, and you've experienced a physical tension or an "atmosphere" in the room. You can't see it but you can *feel it.* What you are feeling is the energy that has come from the thoughts and emotions from those who have been arguing. This energy does two things; firstly it affects the emotions and behaviour of other people it comes in contact with. In the scenario I just mentioned, on entering the room and picking up on this energy, you will in some way respond to it. You might even find that it triggers something in your own past, which causes you to react to the situation, either appropriately or inappropriately. At the very least you are likely to feel uncomfortable or concerned.

Secondly, the law of attraction tells us that this energy attracts back to us more of the same. In the scenario mentioned above, if the couple consistently argue they will attract back to themselves all the fears and negativity that they have expressed, and things get worse.

Emotions also carry different energy levels. For example depression has a different energy level to happiness. Someone suffering from depression has a low energy level which is why they find it so difficult to be motivated, even to do things that they consciously know will make them feel better, whereas someone who is happy has a higher energy level which allows them to feel motivated and interested in life and does fun things with little or no effort.

If you are daily focusing your thoughts, visualising, and affirming your ideal relationship you will create within you a change of energy. You will shift from being negative about the future to feeling positive and motivated, and you will find you have more physical energy and vitality than you previously had. This energy impacts not only on your attitude but also fires you into action, which won't go unnoticed by others. You will find you become interested in new hobbies or activities, you will feel like socialising more, and become more open to making new friends. You will find that like-minded people will become attracted to you, and positive situations will present themselves to you.

All this is great news as it is in your power to bring about. Only you can change the way the feel, but, something else happens too. Your brain will actually start to seek out people whose qualities match the 'blueprint' you have created in your mind. It does this through the reticular activating system (RAS) which is situated at the base of the brain stem. The RAS has many important functions, one of which is to filter all the stimuli that your senses pick up and bring to your conscious attention those things you have an interest in. To give you an example of how information is filtered through your hearing, have you ever had the experience of being in a conversation with someone whilst at a party, and amongst all the noise and music you suddenly pick up on another conversation at the other side of the room which interests you and you tune into it? Suddenly because you heard a specific word that interests you, you become "all ears". That was because your RAS brought it to your attention. So the point I'm making here is, without any effort on your part, your RAS will automatically bring to your attention those things you have trained your subconscious to seek (in the form of your visualisations and affirmations).Isn't that fantastic? So be open to meeting new and interesting people, you never know when your RAS will bring someone to your attention, and who knows, you might find yourself bumping into someone 'accidentally' who turns out to be your ideal partner.

What with the universal law of attraction working positively for you and your own brain quietly seeking out potential partners, your ideal partner will appear, as long as you keep sending out the right vibrational energy each day through visualising, affirming and believing.

The great thing about this is that no longer do you need to be 'desperately seeking', providing you do your daily meditations, and allow your subconscious to do the rest – you will effortlessly find your ideal partner.

Tip # 17 Honour a Place in your Life for a Relationship

"After you wave goodbye to your grieving and complaining about your loss, turn around and look at a new land."- Author unknown

To enjoy a successful and fulfilling relationship you need to create physical space in your life. As well as clearing out the emotional toxins that pollute your chances of meeting the right person, you also need to clear your physical space to make room for love. Start with your living space, and clear out old stuff from previous relationships. I'm talking about the photos you may have lying around of your last relationship, as well as other items or gifts that serve as a reminder to a past love.

Plan to clear out cupboards and rooms and throw out stuff that drains your energy and keeps you stuck in the past. Do this slowly and methodically, gradually working your way through your entire living space, car and if necessary your workspace. Release any emotions that tie you to the past, and work through any pain of loss.

Likewise if you are leading a busy lifestyle with lots of work and personal activities, then you definitely would need to review these in order to create plenty of space for a relationship. Furthermore you could find yourself too busy and miss the opportunity of meeting your life partner. Being in a fulfilling relationship doesn't mean you have to stop being an individual, and it is important you continue with your own personal hobbies and interests, after all, it is your individuality that will attract the right person to you. But remember balance is important, so give serious thought as to how much time you allocate and trim up where necessary, after all you will soon have a new priority in life,

Tip # 18 Honour a Place in your Heart for a Relationship

"Since love grows within you, so beauty grows. For love is the beauty of the soul. " ~ Saint Augustine

To find your ideal partner, or soul mate, is to do more than wish, hope or dream. It requires having an intention and to take the action needed to be sure you attract the right partner into your life. It is necessary to honour a place in your heart for a relationship and be committed not only to personal self-growth and healing, but to a willingness to be open and vulnerable. Opening your heart to another person is not an easy task, especially if you have been hurt in the past and takes courage. However, if you are genuinely yearning to share a deeply intimate, honest relationship with someone, then you need to become willing to receive love, which for some people can be the hardest part. Resist letting feelings of rejection, hurt, or even outrage sour your view of the future.

When you meet someone who could potentially be your ideal partner, give yourself permission to lay down any emotional barriers that stop you from giving love. This shouldn't be overwhelming or suffocating to him/her, but by gently offering genuine care and support. Be an active listener and treat him/her with respect. Love is an unselfish caring about the interests of the other person, often putting their desires before your own. In doing this your will create more space in your heart enabling to receive love back. Remember the more space you release in your heart the more space you'll have to receive.

Tip # 19 Celebrate Your Life

"The more you praise and celebrate your life, the more there is in life to celebrate" – Oprah Winfrey

It's important that wherever you are in life's mysterious journey, enjoy life to the full. Plan and visualize the future but also enjoy the present moment. As for the past, only look back on memories that serve you. Your daily exercises and meditations should only take up 20 or so minutes a day, for the rest of the day enjoy the present as you discover new and exciting opportunities that come your way. Life is an exciting journey and not just a series of goals to be met.

Create a life of pleasure, fun and purpose living each day to the full. Discover how to be complete within yourself. Finding the ideal partner for you is not about having another person to complete you, you are already complete. Inside you are all the resources and help you need, all you have to do is discover them. Love is about two people joining together and sharing and supporting each other in the journey of life. Love should be free and not an obligation to meet another's needs or demands. Nor is it about control and domination.

Remember the most precious gift you have is time – don't waste a moment of it. Relax and go with the flow, confident in the knowledge that the relationship you are attracting will come to you one day, and in the meantime, fill your life with the things you love to do, spending time doing the things that make you feel good.

One of the key things to help us be happy just as we are is acceptance. If we can accept who we are and how life is for us at this moment of time, then we move in gratitude.

So how can we totally accept ourselves and our life as it is? We start by accepting our past, and all that has occurred. That's not having regrets and seeing mistakes and failures as being the perfect lessons for us, essential for our maturity and well-being.

You see, we live in a perfect system, with a perfect order in place. The solar system is perfect, with each planet orbiting the sun. The Earth is perfect, spinning on its axis at exactly the right angle, and speed to sustain a perfect atmosphere, which supports life – animal and vegetation - perfectly.

If these big things have perfect order, then it makes sense to assume so do the little things. Otherwise we would have complete chaos. Everything on our planet is in balance and in harmony with each other. It is perfect. This is why there is so much concern in recent years about mankind's interference with this balance. Yet despite this interference, nature will ultimately win.

Despite mankind's worst efforts, humans cannot interfere with the order within the universe.

This brings me to the point that if you can accept that everything that has happened, and is happening now in your life, good and bad, is perfect for you and essential for you to grow into the person you are meant to be, then your attitude to life, past, present and future changes to one of peace. Look back over your life and identify events that at the time were bad experiences, but later you came to see them as good for you. It could be a broken relationship, or even a health problem, for example a heart attack. These things happened for a reason. Maybe the heart attack led to you making healthier life choices, and that broken relationship will open the door to a loving relationship with a new partner.

Accept and live in gratitude for everything you have and for each day and you will be surprised how your energy level will increase because your attitude to life has changed. Start by keeping a "Gratitude Diary" and write in it each day the achievements and experiences you have each day. It's easy to be grateful for the good things that happen, but allow yourself to be grateful for the not so good things too – there is something to be learnt in all of them that you could be grateful for. Having gratitude means having a great attitude to life, which attracts even more blessings.

Remember whilst you are focusing and expressing the positives in life, more of the same will come back to you. You'll be a great person to be around and an encouragement and strength to others.

Tip # 20 Take Time to Check Out

"You have to walk carefully in the beginning of love; the running across fields into your lovers arms can only come later when your sure they won't laugh if you trip"

- Source Unknown

True love can never be hurt by time. I may be old fashioned, but there is great strength in spending time getting to know someone fully before you fully commit to a life-long relationship. And any commitment you do make should be with your eyes wide open.

One of the dangers during the romantic love stage is that if you are not careful, you can get easily caught up in the overpowering emotion, and overlook good judgement. In other words, just because a gift is wrapped perfectly in glittering paper, remember it tells you nothing about what's inside.

Furthermore, because of your desire to be loved, don't allow yourself to be pushed into a sexual relationship before you are ready to. You run the risk of being emotionally hurt, rejected or manipulated into a damaging relationship, and your emotions will cloud your judgement further. In showing self-control you will get to know their secret heart before you commit to an intimate relationship.

Instead enjoy taking things slowly. During this period you'll be subconsciously and consciously checking out whether this person is someone you can trust and respect, and right for you in a long-term relationship.

When you first meet someone, it is hard to 'see' their personality, to do so you will need to find out their thoughts, hopes, fears, plans, habits and skills, which takes time. When you first meet someone you only see their outer shell and what they want you to see. Giving yourself time to get to know them will enable you to crack the shell and get to the person underneath. Asking open-ended questions is a great way to flush out the real person, enabling you to check out their values to see if they're similar to yours. An example of this would be "if money was no object what would you like to do with your life". You may be surprised by their answers.

Asking questions is a great way of finding more about a person, and will assist you in forming an opinion of whether your values are compatible and will give you insight on how he or she feels about you.

Spending time with someone before forming a commitment allows you the opportunity to get to know how she or he responds to all kinds of situations, seeing them at their "best" and at their "worst". So make sure you plan activities that include "ordinary" every day things and not just dinner dates or trips out somewhere together. This will help you explore their behaviour in different scenarios. Remember I said earlier that people will consistently be who they are, so sooner or later you will discover the REAL person under the outer image. Unpleasant habits and tendencies will reveal themselves to you and will play a role in your decision to commit or not to this person.

Love is unselfish, kind and respectful, so ask yourself these questions:

"Does this person tend to put me down or build me up?"

"Is he/she eager for the success of my achievements and plans or only for his or her own?"

"Does he or she show respect for my views and my feelings".

All relationships are gifts, and give living feedback to us for our own self-growth. Taking time to get to know someone also gives you the opportunity to respond to their feedback and work on your inner self.

So don't be in a rush. Real love doesn't happen overnight, give your relationship time to blossom.

Tip # 21 Know the Difference between Real Love and Infatuation

"Love is what is left in a relationship after all the selfishness is taken out."

- Nick Richardson

How do you know whether what you are feeling is love, or whether it is infatuation? First of all we need a definition of love. Love is an unselfish caring about the interests of another, where you want to give and share with the other person, putting your own wants as secondary. You are attracted by the other person's total personality and their spiritual qualities, and not blind to their faults. When you are in love you respect the other person, you are patient and kind and take time to resolve disagreements amicably taking into account the other persons perspective.

Whereas infatuation is the opposite, infatuation is selfish and restrictive. The appearance of the other person is paramount, and because of this, he or she seems perfect to you. You ignore and reject any nagging doubts that you may have about serious personality flaws. The emphasis is about self-satisfaction, particularly with regard to sex, and any arguments you may have are rarely resolved and glossed over by a kiss.

In following all the guidance in this booklet you will have developed a sense of what love looks like. You will have learnt to see through your own spiritual eyes and will have a clearer understanding of who you are. You will have a deep sense of knowing or a "gut feeling" or even a small voice in your head guiding you, and by getting in touch with your internal guidance, you will be able to access and listen to the voice of wisdom in your choice of partner.

If you know yourself fully, you can trust your intuition or inner wisdom, and you will simply 'know' when he or she turns up in your life.

Workshops Run by Fast Forward Therapies

'Heart Matters'

Couples 7- day workshop at La Platriere Retreat, France

This couple's workshop is a journey for every couple who wants to gain insight into how you can create a deeply satisfying and long-lasting relationship with your partner. It's not only ideal for couples who have just met, but also for those couples who are struggling in their relationship, as it assists you both in understanding what inevitably occurs in a relationship, and teaches you the skills in dealing with problems.

This transformational workshop takes place in an idyllic setting, at La Platriere, in the Auvergne, in France, where you'll not only receive new learning, but will be able to explore the region. La Platriere, situated on a hill with stunning views of surrounding countryside, is a tranquil, healing place where time stands still. The area has been unchanged for many years, and is unspoilt by tourism, and far from the madding crowds, with fortresses and chateaux, medieval villages and festivals, forests and lakes, French markets and thermal spas, La Platriere is surrounded by beauty.

Visit www.fastforwardtherapies.co.uk for full details or email Jackie on jackie@fastforwardtherapies.co.uk

Workshops Run by Jackie Hill
Living a Purpose Led Life

Do you feel life has no purpose and every day is just the same?"

"Are you a victim of life's circumstance and accident, being tossed this way and that?"

"Do you feel that life is a game of chance, a series of good and bad luck, depending on whether you are in the right place at the right time?

If you've answered yes to any of these 3 questions; then I have some really good news for you!

If I told you, you were born with a life purpose, a reason for your very existence, and by fulfilling this purpose you would feel joy, have a sense of direction, and create an interesting life
And that I could show you how to discover that purpose? Would you want to know how?

If I told you, you could live a life whereby you felt in control, that you could develop a road map of where you wanted to go, and discover the "how" of getting there – would you be interested to know more?

If I told you that your energy is a magnet within the universe, that you attract positive or negative vibrations to your life depending on what you think and feel, and taught you how to benefit from this

Law of Attraction to manifest the good things in life you desire – would you want that?

If the answer is YES...

Then join me at La Platriere in France for your journey of discovering who you are and how to achieve the life you're meant to life.

Start "Living the Purpose Led Life"

Visit www.fastforwardtherapies.co.uk for full details or email Jackie on jackie@fastforwardtherapies.co.uk

Practical Resources

Hypnotherapy:

The School of Analytical and Cognitive Hypnotherapy (SACH) for lists of therapists; www.sachinternational.com

The General Hypnotherapy Register for therapists in your area: www.general-hypnotherapy-register.co,

The British Hypnotherapy Association: www.bhahynotherapy.org

Counselling

Look in your local telephone directory for counselors close to you or checkout on the internet.

About Jackie Hill

Jackie Hill has many years experience as an integrative psychotherapist, clinical hypnotherapist, and NLP practitioner. She has helped many people over the years working with individuals, families and couple relationship counselling. She ran a successful private practice Fast Forward Therapies Ltd in Suffolk for several years, and now works from La Platriere Retreat in France which she runs with her husband.

Jackie is the owner of Fast Forward UK based in France. She teaches self-growth workshops, as well as running relationship workshops and de-stress weekends in France. She offers life-coaching and counselling sessions and has developed a successful residential 4-7 days smoking cessation programme at La Platriere.

For more information about any of the above or about any of the information products she has made on self-improvement such as books, workbooks, CDs, MP3 downloads, and DVDs please visit her website www.fastforwardtherapies.co.uk. You can also subscribe to Jackie's free newsletter, which will keep you updated with new events and promotions and special offers as well handy tips and advice on personal growth, please contact Jackie by email through the Fast Forward website.